NUTRITION
BARNEY STYLE

Jordan R. Bennefeld

ISBN-13: 978-1973832799

CONTENTS

DEDICATION

This book is dedicated to anyone who puts forth the time and effort to better themselves. No one can put forth the effort for us. It comes from within.

INTRO

STOP BULLSHITTIN'

Let's start this thing off right, because I don't want anyone to get the wrong impression. This isn't a "Get fit in 2 weeks" type of book, nor am I going to tell you about a magic pill. There isn't a secret that only fit people know about and there is no shortcut to getting a swole ass body.

However, there are a few things that will help you reach your goal. Here is a few: Hard work, discipline, effort, sacrifice, dedication, will power, persistence. Should I go on, or do you get my point?

Stop lying to yourself about wanting to change your eating habits or going to the gym more. If you really wanted that shit bad enough, you would've already started.

Then I hear about the whole, "New year new me" crock of shit. I HATE hearing that excuse. The only thing that is, is a way for you to buy more time before you actually start putting in the work. And 9 times out of 10, it will last a max of a few months before you start telling yourself that, "Next year will be MY year!"

Stop bullshittin' yourself. Since when do we need a fucking date to better ourselves? Why not today, tonight, right now, before work, after work? If you really want something bad enough, you will start right now. Stop making excuses for yourself just to buy more time to be lazy and complacent.

Now that we got that out of the way, this book is mainly focused on nutrition. With nutrition comes exercise, so I'll touch on that as well with each section. I say nutrition because sometimes the word "diet" gets confusing to people. When I say diet, I simply mean the stuff you put into your body. No I don't mean those new beads you just bought, I mean food, drink, supplements, anything that you ingest for nutrition.

Some people hear the word diet and think about 2 weeks of no soda and no bread. Or they think about starving themselves just because they have a wedding or pool party coming up. I have 2 words for that, fuck that. Those results are only temporary and starving your body is not the way to get in shape.

If you want long-term results that will last, you have to change your whole damn lifestyle. This isn't something you do for a month and then think you can stop, this is something, if you want it bad enough, that you will instill into yourself and change your ways. Habits are ok if they are good habits.

A short summary to live an overall better, healthier life – drink water, eat veggies, eat lean meat, and workout. That is basically the key to being fit in a nutshell. Obviously there are a lot more aspects that you can take into consideration, if not this would be the end of the book.

CHAPTER 1

MINDSET

If you're wanting to do this because you love food, you're wrong. You have to change the way you think. We don't do it for the flavor, we do it for the fuel. This isn't a health kick or just a phase, this shit is a lifestyle. Either you have it in you or you don't.

Now yes, there are numerous ways you can go about this lifestyle and still eat some pretty good food, that's why I have included some recipes. But the main focus is not going to be how good your meal is. Your focus needs to be when your next feeding is. You think lions kill their prey then try to find some salt and a nice wine to pair with it? Fuck no. They eat that shit because they're a beast and that's what beasts do.

Life is all about decisions. Everything you do is a decision and the results will depend on that decision. I don't want to hear any damn excuses about how your wife only cooks fried food and you have no choice. Eat something else. Don't grab the fucking cookie, grab a carrot and eat that instead. I hate when people try to blame their environment on their life. You have the ability to change those things.

Next time you go to the grocery store, don't buy junk shit. Buy your produce, your proteins, and other essentials. Oreos is not an essential.

Now you already should know what I'm about to say next...EVERYONE IS DIFFERENT! So you need to find a meal plan that works for you.

Find Your Why:

Why? Why do YOU want to change? Someone can tell you that it's healthier or that you will look more fit, but why do you want this? You need to dig deep and figure out what is it that pushed you to buy this book or that thing that constantly pops into your head that drives you towards a better lifestyle. Is it for looks, is it for your kids, is it for health? You decide. But whatever it is, you need to eat, sleep, and breath it in order to accomplish it. Half assed effort will give you half assed results.

Determine a Goal:

What is it that you're wanting to accomplish? What do you want your end result to be? Are you looking to bulk, cut, get toned, lose fat? Depending on your answer will determine the steps that you need to take to get there. Every plan is custom to you and your goal.

Make a Plan:

Now that you know what you want and why you want it, it's time to prepare for it. I'm going to guide you with this part, but again, everything is going to be custom to what works for you. So I will give you a basic foundation, then you tweak it from there. You need to determine how you're going to go about doing it, you're schedule, and execute.

Execute:

Execute the things that you have planned to do. You know what you want to do, why you want to do it, and how you want to do it. Now you need to do it. Don't slack on execution when you have a written out plan. You just need to suck it up and do what it takes to get to your goal, then demolish that goal.

CHAPTER 2

THE BASICS

Everything starts with a good foundation. Like my Bodybuilding book, it is the basic essentials to build a good foundation to build on. Nutrition is no different. You want to lay the basic groundwork to build a solid foundation in order for you to maintain a healthy body.

Before I get into anything else, water. Drink it. Drink plenty of it. Water water water. For those of you that ARE looking for a quick, easy out, a little fun fact is that if you drink a gallon of water for a week, you can lose up to 10 lbs. Most of us retain water because we don't drink enough of it. Sounds stupid, I know, but stop thinking and keep reading.

Our bodies retain water when we don't

get enough. Think of it as survival mode. It is going to hang onto and store every drop because it isn't sure when it will get more. By drinking more water, your body now knows that it gets a constant and regular supply. Therefore, it will flush out water and not store it because it is getting more. So if you want to lose water weight, drink more of it.

Our bodies use water in the cells, organs, and tissues to help regulate temperature and maintain bodily functions. The human body is about 65% water and our muscles need to stay hydrated in order to grow. The less water we have, the more dehydratedour muscles and organs get, the less gains we get. No one wants less gains.

As for food, first and foremost, vegetables. You can never ever ever get enough of them. Rule of thumb, green is great. Anything green is packed with nutrients and vitamins that are essential to your body. Broccoli, kale, green beans, spinach, etc. That's not to say that other vegetables are bad, because they are all great, for the most part. So don't neglect carrots, squash, zucchini, etc.

Now, not the get too hipster on you, but juicing is a great way to get your daily intake of veggies. Throw in some cucumbers, kale, carrots, and slam it down. Juicing is a great way to get some energy in the morning or before a workout. I'm not implying that you go on a juice cleanse or anything, I'm merely suggesting that putting it into your diet as an addition can be beneficial.

Another thing is how and when you eat veggies that determine how beneficial they are. What I do, is when eating my meal, I tend to eat most of my veggies first. I do this for 2 reasons.

The first is to get them out of the way. I personally like vegetables, but if you aren't too keen on them, go ahead and scarf them down to get them out of the way. The second reason is to get them into your body first. If you have an empty stomach, your body is in need of substance and is looking for food. If you throw all those veggies in there, it will start processing them right away and taking advantage of all the nutrients.

The same goes on the flipside to all this. If the first thing you put into your body is potato chips, your body will start absorbing everything it can from them. I think we can both agree that we would rather our bodies take advantage of greens instead of Doritos.

Real quick, while we're on the subject of Doritos, I know they taste great, this is not a mystery. But again, if you are serious about this, you need to understand that we aren't doing this for the taste, we do it for the fuel. When I was in Marine Corps boot camp, we had to eat as fast as we could. Our Drill Instructors would constantly yell at us, "Hurry up, you're not eating for the flavor!"

Now don't get me wrong, no one enjoys eating bland, boring, food. That is where I got your back. Later on we'll discuss how to prepare food, as well as a few recipes so that you can actually enjoy eating healthy.

Enough of that, next we have our protein. A common rule of thumb for protein is to eat 1 gram of protein for every pound of body weight. That is a basic rule to live by. If you're bulking, you will bump that up to 1.5 or 2 grams per pound.

Keep in mind, more protein does not mean more muscle. Your body can only take in so much. Excessive protein intake can result in unwanted weight gain, dehydration, and stress on your kidneys. More than enough simply converts to extra calories, into sugar, and then fat. So to make things simple, eating too much protein will make you an unhealthy fat ass. Everyone is different and reacts differently though, so find out what works best for you.

Types of good protein consist mainly of lean meat. Chicken, fish, turkey, and a little red meat is the common foundation. To get a perspective, here is the protein content for a few: Lean chicken breast (31g for 3.5oz), salmon (30g for 5oz), tuna (25g 3oz), Ribeye (69g for 10oz).

Now, you may look at this and think, "Damn, looks like I'm going on a ribeye diet." False. Check yo-self. That is a 10oz steak for starters, and while the ribeye has one of the highest protein contents, it is also filled with bad fat and red meat also contains cholesterol. I try to keep my red meat intake to about once a week or less.

One of the best options is actually the salmon. It may not have as much protein as the ribeye or chicken titty, but it offers more, such as omega 3 fatty acids that are extremely beneficial. If you aren't taking omega-3 everyday, you're wrong. You can buy fish oil, that contains omega-3, anywhere vitamins are sold. Omega-3 helps with muscle growth, metabolism, anti-depression, focus, energy, literally everything that is good. Take that shit.

Chicken breast is probably one of the most common choices for those who want to stay away from red meat and don't care for fish. You can bake it, sear it, grill it, boil it, whatever you want to do. Cut the fat off and go to down for some good, lean protein. Chicken gets pretty old to the palate, but remember, we're doing this for the gains, not the taste.

Now for foods that are great in protein, but aren't meats, I introduce you to black beans. This is probably one of my favorites. It goes well with any food and taste great. A cup of black beans contains 15g of protein and about 15g of fiber. You can't go wrong with that. Personally, I can easily eat about 2 cups in one sitting.

Another great source of protein is quinoa (keen-wah). It's more than just hipster bird food. While it is commonly mistaken for a grain, quinoa is actually a seed. 1 cup of cooked quinoa has a little over 8 grams of protein. That is less that the black beans, but quinoa is considered a complete protein. That means that you are getting all 9 essential amino acids into your body. The best part about quinoa is that it can be eaten in place of carbs. While it's not a carb, it will help ease your carb cravings.

To put things into perspective, I am 250lbs. A normal meal for me is 1/2 lb of chicken breast, a cup of black beans, and a cup of quinoa. That alone is around 90 grams of protein. That is almost 1/3 of my suggested protein intake, in one meal. I usually eat about 5 eggs in the morning, which is roughly around 30g. So breakfast and lunch will put me right around the halfway mark. A big dinner, some lean snacks, and a protein shake will put me right where I need to be.

Carbs. Everyone is scared of the carbs. Carbs are needed for energy. If you are going to live an active and healthy lifestyle, you need carbs. Unless you're cutting for a show, carbs will be a part of your nutrition. Now, excess carbs is where the problems begin.

The body uses carbs as energy. You may have played sports and have heard the term "carb loading." That's where the night before a big game, you eat a shit ton of pasta to carb load. The reason for this is to have excess energy for that big game. It works in this scenario because you will burn and use the carbs. If you just eat a giant bowl of pasta and sit on your ass the whole day, you're probably going to feel like shit.

When you regularly eat excessive amounts of carbs, your body will not only gain weight, but it will store fewer carbs in the cells as energy. The rest of those carbs get processed through your body, ultimately becoming fat.

When you eat carbs matters. Eating carbs in the morning is ok because you will use and burn them throughout the day.

Same goes for lunch, you will use and burn them at the gym. However, I try to avoid carbs for dinner. This is because you are not active at night. So if you put all these carbs into your body, then go to sleep, you're not going to burn nearly as many. Unless you're carb loading for a marathon or some shit, but even then, you don't do that every day.

Veggies, fruits, and beans contain carbs, but they are not starches. Starchy carbs are the ones you need to be mindful about, bread, pasta, white rice, potatoes. They are high in refined sugar and turn into fat. Too much sugar can cause metabolic dysfunction, which can result in weight gain, abdominal obesity, as well as elevated blood sugar and blood pressure.

With all this sugar talk, let's get into fruits. While we grew up thinking that fruits are good for us, they are for the most part, but the downfall is the sugar They contain tons of vitamins that are essential. If you want to eat an orange or banana or apple as a snack, go for it. I just don't recommend eating a shit ton of fruit on a daily basis. However, eating a couple pieces of fruit can be beneficial before a workout.

A small rule that I go by, is shopping the perimeter of the grocery store. That is where you will find the majority of the food you need. All of your meats, poultry, eggs, milk, veggies, fruit, is all on the perimeter.

Overall, you just need to keep shit real with yourself. You know what's good and what isn't good for you. Don't try to convince yourself that you can eat cake just because you took the icing off. Don't feel good about yourself just because you drank 2 bottles of water and had a salad that consisted of mostly ranch.

That is the beauty of fitness, you cannot cheat and get away with it. The only person you're lying to is yourself. I don't give a shit if you tell me that you ate clean for 6 months, the fact that you're out of breath walking up one flight of stairs and your sweat smells like beef broth gives you away.

Above all, I don't give a shit if you get in shape or not. It's your goal, not mine. But if you want to be able to live a long, healthy life and be able to play with your kids without having a heart attack, I suggest you take a little initiative and get your shit together. You don't have to be a yoga, hipster, health nut, you just have to be mindful of the things that you're putting into your body.

To get an idea of foods that are good for you, here is a list of acceptable foods:

Proteins:

Tilapia	Eggs
Salmon	Tuna
Shrimp	Lean steak
Chicken breast	Turkey breast
Quinoa	Black beans

Vegetables:

Green beans	Cucumber
Broccoli	Mushrooms
Cauliflower	Bell Pepper
Kale	Brussel sprouts
Spinach	Onions
Romaine	Beets
Squash	Radishes
Zucchini	Celery
Cabbage	

Fruit:

Green apples	Blueberries
Oranges	Peaches
Watermelon	Plums
Strawberries	Tomatoes
Red grapes	Cherries
Grapefruit	Cantaloupe
Kiwi	Banana

Carbs:

Sweet potatoes	Brown Rice
Bananas	Whole wheat pasta
Beans	Oatmeal
Pumpkin	Butternut squash
Whole wheat pasta	Peas

Good Fats:

Avocado	Natural peanut butter
Olive Oil	Light Mayo
Light Mayo	Light butter
Nuts	Olives
Flaxseed	Edamame
Sunflower seeds	Yogurt

A Few Good Snacks:

Rice cakes	Nuts
Greek Yogurt	Raisins
Almonds	Edamame
Banana	

CHAPTER 3

BULKING

People ask all the time, "How do you get big?" The answer is simple, if you want to get big, you have to eat big. Bulking is where the weight comes on. The method is to eat tons of calories and intake to build massive amounts of muscle. Then you cut the fat off and are left with lean muscle.

Well, some people tend to take this shit a little too far. I always joke around and say that I bulk 24/7/365, but in a reality, I just eat somewhat-clean with a lot of protein. Some people think they can eat whatever the fuck they want and lift heavy shit in order to achieve this. We call this "Dirty Bulking."

Dirty bulking works for individuals who were born with that thing called metabolism. They can eat a shit ton of pizza and fried chicken, workout, and burn it off. Overall, that's not the healthiest approach you want to take.

When I'm in "bulking mode" I tend to cheat more often, but I do it with stuff like homemade double-cheeseburgers with lean beef. I may get down on a big ass turkey leg or eat a pizza the night before deadlift day, but I keep these type of meals minimal, maybe once a week.

Just don't eat dirty ALL THE TIME. Bulking doesn't mean free will to eat whatever the fuck you want. You want to eat plenty of protein, plenty of carbs, and good fats. You're only eating this much because you are tearing shit up in the gym and making the weights your bitch. When it's bulking time, you are giving it 197% in the gym every time.

Let's be clear about this, if you eat like you're bulking, but don't workout like you're bulking, you will get fat.

Your body and your muscles need fuel to keep trucking, so you have to shovel that shit in and feed them. The best time to bulk is after dieting and eating clean for a while. This way, your body will soak everything up like a sponge.

You want to up your protein intake from 1g per lb of body weight to about 1.5g to 2g per lb. This will give you the extra protein your muscles need to grow. For carbs, you want to take in about 1.5 – 2g per lb of body weight. All the extra carbs will supply you with the energy needed to be a fucking beast.

Again, when you consume certain things also plays a role. You want to have your carbs mainly in the morning and post-workout. Try to avoid carbs later in the evening as you will be less likely to burn them off. For your protein, you want it split up evenly throughout the day, which means more meals. Instead of the traditional 3 meals a day, try to split it up into 6 smaller meals. This will provide your body with a constant supply and it will use it more efficiently.

You will still need to drink plenty of water. Water. Water. Water. You should be drinking at least a gallon a day. I'm a milk drinker, so you can drink milk as well. Whole milk with give you more fats, but if you choose to do 2% (watered-down milk) that's ok too. As always, try to avoid soda and sports drinks. If you have one every once in a while, you won't die, but just don't make it a habit. Same goes for beer…

What is bulking if you don't put it to use? It's just extra weight if you don't use it. Again, you will gain some fat in this process, but the main result is gaining more muscle mass. Therefore, training is paramount. If you're not going to skip out on meals, then don't skip out on the weights.

You can stick with your regular training, such as chest on Mondays, arms on Tuesdays, back on Wednesdays, and legs on Thursdays, or however you train. But the main thing is to go harder and heavier. We're not shooting for the beach body, Spartan 300, Magic Mike body just yet. Right now we're focused on the night club security, hulk, defensive lineman body.

A routine that I typically stick with, and I talk about in my Bodybuilding book, is doing more sets and more reps. This style of lifting will give you results, but for bulking, we want to up the weight and lower the reps just a tad. Usually I do anywhere from 8 to 12 sets at about 12 to

20 reps. Keep in mind, this is usually done at a good medium weight. We want to up it to a medium/heavy weight, doing about 5 to 8 sets at about 10 to 12 reps. If you're able to do 15 to 18 reps per set, then you're not going heavy enough. Quit being a bitch and add some more plates.

Now we're really digging deep and tearing those muscle fibers up. The idea is to think big! I talk about visualizing yourself being a massive beast and having that intense mind/muscle connection. Don't just go through the motions and movements. You need to execute properly and engage in whatever muscle you're training.

The Big 3 will play a huge role in the bulking process. That is: Bench, Squat, Deadlift. These 3 exercises will give you an, overall, solid core and foundation. You're hitting the big muscle groups that will increase strength and testosterone to give you those massive gains.

A rough idea of what a bulking cycle would be like goes like this:

Breakfast: 5 eggs and 2 pieces toast.

2nd Breakfast: oatmeal and a protein shake.

Lunch: Chicken breast, cup of brown rice, cup of veggies.

2nd Lunch: Protein shake and a banana.

Dinner: Ribeye and a ton of veggies.

Midnight Snack: protein shake.

For working out:

Monday: Chest. Heavy weights, lots of bench, 6 sets, 10-12 reps.

Tuesday: Legs. Medium to heavy weight. Lots of squats and leg presses, 8 sets, 10-12 reps.

Wednesday: Back. Medium to heavy weight, lots and lots of deadlifts. 6-8 sets, 8-10 reps.

Thursday: Arms. Lots of shoulders and triceps. Medium on the shoulders and heavy on the tris. 6-8 sets and 10-12 reps.

Friday: Either have an off day or do chest again.

You want to train about 4-6 times a week. Again, everyone is different, so choose what works best for you. I typically train about 5 to 6 days a week with 1 or 2 off days thrown in the mix. I try not to have my off days back-to-back, but every few weeks I will just to give my body rest.

It's also important to rest in between sets more. With bulking, you want to let the muscles get plenty of oxygen and blood flow before pushing them again. So I recommend about 2-3 minutes in between sets, especially since you'll be lifting a lot heavier.

Speaking of rest, sleep is very crucial in the bulking process. You want to get plenty of rest to let your body heal from all the hard lifting and training that you have been putting it through. A solid 8 hours of sleep every night is critical. If you are able to, take hour naps throughout the day if you feel you need the extra rest.

I am usually against scales because, personally, I don't care what I weigh. I just go off of what I look like and how much weight I am lifting. But for bulking, you may want to hop on a scale at least once a week. This is so you know if you need to up your food intake or not.

If you weigh 200 lbs on week 1 and now it's week 3 and you only weight 203, something ain't right. If you are 3 weeks in on a serious bulking cycle, you should be somewhere around 210 mark, at LEAST. Again, everyone is different, so track yourself. Professional bodybuilders can put on tons of weight in a short period of time, but their food intake is astronomical.

How long should you bulk? It takes some time to get the desired results, so you can't bulk for a week then cut for a week and so on. That's just stupid. Realistically, you want to run a program for about 10 to 12 weeks. This will give you plenty of time to make the necessary changes to your body.

A successful bulking cycle can put on

anywhere from 20 to 40 pounds, with about 80% of that being muscle. Some people are able to put on more and some people less. For the 87th time, everyone is different. After bulking comes the cutting, where we shed that fat and still maintain most of the muscle.

CHAPTER 4

CUTTING

Cutting is where the hard work and effort of bulking show through. But on the flipside to the glory comes sacrifice. Bulking was the fun part of eating all the time and lifting heavy shit. Now we get to cut back on everything and lift for reps.

Everyone likes the idea of cutting and getting ripped and shredded, but it's not until they find out how it's done that they quickly turn away from it. Personally, the shit sucks. I don't ever really do a true cutting phase. I just go through a bulking stage then I clean up my diet and lift a little differently.

There are tons of theories, philosophies, methods, and ways you can go about this. Some people count this and cut that and blah blah blah. Fuck all that. This is a basic guide.

Some people regard cutting as simply losing fat to get a little lean, while others regard it as getting ready for a show. In which case, they count ounces of stuff like water and count every little gram of carbs and protein. It takes a lot of discipline to achieve that, but if you've ever seen a show, the results pay off.

Well this shit is Barney Style kid. So we're going to go through a basic plan for a cutting cycle.

You know all those delicious meals and all that food you were eating? Yea, well that shit is coming to a halt. It's time to cut back on the calories. That means a little on the protein and cut back on the carbs.

As mentioned before with bulking, we wanted to eat as much as possible to fuel our muscles. Our main goal was to gain size in muscles. Well now that we have increased our muscle mass, our main goal is to shed the fat so that all the hard work can show. So with cutting, we are removing the fat layer, which is a byproduct of bulking.

We want to burn off more calories than we take in. Now, we were consuming about 1.5g of protein per lb of bodyweight. We're going to cut that back to 1 for 1. This will lower our caloric intake and help us to lose some of that unwanted weight. For carbs, we're going to do about 1-1.5g per lb of bodyweight, maybe even less. We still need carbs, but this way, we will burn through them and start using our 2nd source of energy, which is fat.

Our main source of protein is going to be chicken breast, turkey, and fish. We want light and lean proteins. Red meat has higher fat content and takes longer to digest. I recommend chicken, lean turkey (93%), tilapia, salmon, and tuna.

Veggies. We need lots of veggies. A lot of the meals will consist mainly of a protein and a vegetable. Broccoli, green beans, squash, are all good choices that we can use. Remember, green is good.

For carbs, we're staying away from all starches such as pastas, bread, white rice, and anything that's processed. We will get a lot of our carbs from brown rice, oatmeal, and a little fruit, like bananas.

You will feel leaner just after a couple weeks of eating this way. Fish, turkey, and chicken tend to digest rather quickly. Not having any starchy foods or unnecessary sugar will make you feel a lot better after meals. Ever notice how after you eat a shit ton of pizza or a big ass hamburger, you just want to lay down and die somewhere?

Eating leaner and lighter will alleviate that.

Here is what a rough outline of daily meals looks like:

Breakfast: 5 egg whites, cup of oatmeal.

2nd Breakfast: Rice cakes

Lunch: 2 cans of tuna, ½ cup of brown rice.

Post-Lunch: Cup of veggies

Dinner: Salmon and lots of veggies

Midnight Snack: Protein shake. Preferably with a protein powder that is lean or low fat.

Again, this is merely an example. For some of you , it may be hard to cut back on the carbs. Tough shit. That is how we cut. No french-fries or tater tots anymore.

The carbs we eat come from brown rice and bananas. But you can always mix things up with different proteins and veggies with the list provided earlier in the 1st chapter.

Our workouts are going to go back to high sets and high reps. This is because we're trying to burn the fat and work the shit out of the muscles. Cardio will also come into play. I know, I hate it too, but if you find a type of cardio that works for you, you can enjoy it more than just hopping on a treadmill. Obstacle courses and circuits work for me.

The workout plan will look similar to the bulking one, except we will adjust the sets and reps and add in the cardio. We still want to train about 5 to 6 days a week, but with our clean diet and the faster paced workouts, we will start to notice a difference within a few weeks.

Monday: 15 mins of stair stepper. Chest. Light to medium weights, flyes and dumbbells, 10 sets, 12-15 reps. End with 15 mins of cardio.

Tuesday: Legs. Medium weight. Lots of squats, leg curls and extensions, 10 sets, 12-15 reps. 15 mins stair stepper.

Wednesday: 15 mins stair stepper. Back. Light to medium weight, lots and lots of deadlifts. 8-10 sets, 12-15 reps.

Thursday: 45 mins cardio

Friday: Arms. Light to medium weight. Hit everything, shoulders, biceps, and triceps. 10-12 sets and 12-20 reps. 15 mins stair stepper.

Remember to incorporate your off day(s) however you see fit. Notice how we threw in cardio almost every day then had a full day of strictly cardio. Also, you want to cut down on your rest periods between sets. Cut it down to about 1-2 mins in between. This way it will keep your heart rate up and burn more calories.

For cardio, I recommend the stair stepper. The idea isn't to sprint, but it's not to be a sloth either. I usually have the speed set around 6 or 7. It is a good speed that compares to a brisk walk, I suppose.

Keep this routine up for about the first 6 to 8 weeks and adjust as needed. The closer you get to the 10 and 12 week mark, cut back on the carbs some more and keep your workouts light, but intense. It is amazing the difference you will see in just a few weeks. Your skin will become tight and all the muscle you put on from your bulk will finally show through.

Once winter comes back around, it's time to do it all over again. Bulk and cut, bulk and cut. It's a repeated process over and over as you continue to build. Just like muscles, you break em down then they build up, over and over.

Each time you go through a cycle, find out what worked for you or what didn't work for you. I can't stress this enough, but everyone is different. Some people get better results with more carbs and less protein or vice versa. So figure it out, but never lose the intensity.

CHAPTER 5

SUPPLEMENTS

Sup-ple-ment: 1. Something that completes or enhances something else when added to it. 2. Add an element or amount to.

You see them everywhere, supplements for this, supplements for that. Pre-workouts, proteins, BCAAs, creatine, blah blah blah. Supplements are made to do just that, supplement.

Too often, I see guys and gals with duffle bags full of pills and powders for this and for that. It almost seems like their diet consists of supplements. Now, don't get me wrong, supplements are very useful, but they should never be used to replace the number one "supplement" of all time, food.

People will say things like, "I've been working out, but I'm not getting any bigger. Should I take protein?" Well, I don't know. What does your diet look like? There are so many other factors that need to be looked at, with diet being number one.

You can't just throw a supplement into the mix and think that it's going to be the answer. And if you do decide to get a supplement, you need familiarize yourself with the ingredients and understand what they do.

With so many supplements on the market today, it's hard to determine what is in them without looking on the back. In my opinion, if it says "Proprietary Blend", stay away from it. You have no clue what that blend consists of and it could just be filler garbage in the first place. Proprietary blends are an easy way for companies to make more of a specific supplement by cutting it with a bunch of useless powder.

I'll go over some popular supplements and talk about what is in each of them, and what each of those ingredients is for.

Pre-Workout

Pre-workouts are made just for that, to take before you work out. They provide you with energy and get your blood pumping in order to have a bat-shit crazy, intense workout. Listed below are common ingredients and what each one of them is used for.

Beta-Alanine: Reduce lactic acid in the muscles. Supplementation of Beta-Alanine has been shown to increase carnosine levels, which can reduce the acidity in working muscles during workouts. Average dosage, 1.5g/serving.

L-Citrulline Malate: Strength, endurance, pump. This is an amino acid normally made by the body. L-Citrulline is converted into L-Arginine, which improves blood flow by creating nitric oxcide (NO), which expands blood vessels. Average dosage, 1g/serving.

Arginine Alpha Ketoglutarate (AAKG): AAKG contains the essential amino acid, L-Arginine. This is important and essential for efficient metabolism of amino acids. This also accommodates the production of energy. Overall, this assists with muscle growth and circulation. Average dosage, 1g/serving.

Caffeine: Most of us know that caffeine helps us with energy. It is a natural stimulant that gives us that pick-me-up. Caffeine is also highly thermogenic and assists with burning fat. It can also help with mental focus and concentration.

Average dosage, 250mg/serving.

Niacin: Niacin, or Vitamin B3, can improve cholesterol levels and lower cardiovascular risks. Niacin is also a thermogenic that assists in burning fat. It helps the body convert carbohydrates into fuel, which the body uses to produce energy. This is the "tingling" sensation you get when you take your pre-workout and will also help with vascularity. Average dosage, 30mg/serving.

Creatine Monohydrate: Similar to protein, it is a nitrogen-containing compound. Creatine is most effective in high-intensity training. It is an osmotically active substance which pulls water into your muscle cells, which increases protein synthesis. Overall, creatine will assist with muscle growth. Average dosage, 2g/serving.

Whey Protein

Protein is what all the guys who want to get big talk about. Delivering your body a constant supply of protein is essential for optimum muscle growth. Protein is made up of amino acids, which are the building blocks of your muscles and body. Without them, it would be impossible to build, repair, or even maintain muscle tissue.

When you workout, you tear your muscle fibers and break them down. When you are done, your body repairs or replaces the broken fibers through a cellular process where it fuses the muscle fibers together. As your muscle fibers get broken down and repaired, they grow thicker to create more muscle, known as muscle hypertrophy.

A typical scoop of protein powder is between 30 and 50 grams, but the calorie count depends on which brand you take.

Typically it is about 100-120 calories. This is to be used to supplement your protein intake, not to be used as a main source.

Branched Chain Amino Acids (BCAA)

BCAAs are made up of 3 essential aminos: Leucine, isoleucine, and valine. They are essential because the body cannot make them out of other amino acids. Therefore, they must be ingested through food or supplements.

A large proportion of our cells, muscles and tissue is made up of amino acids, meaning they carry out many important bodily functions, such as giving cells their structure.

There are 20 amino acids in the body, but the 3 provides from BCAAs are the key amino acids that stimulate protein synthesis.

These are 3 of the most common supplements that are taken: pre-workout, protein, and BCAAs. There are plenty more out there that say they do different things. Choose your supplements wisely, but don't rely only on them. You need to make sure that your diet is in check before and while taking supplements.

Also, keep in mind that just because your favorite bodybuilder is in a magazine holding a bottle of pills or powder, doesn't mean it is legit. They do it for the money. Often times, there are guys who promote supplements, but don't even take them themselves. Again, they do it for the paycheck.

If you are interested in a supplement, take the time to look at the supplement facts and research the ingredients in it. This way, you will know what the ingredients actually do, but more importantly, you will know what you are putting into your body.

CHAPTER 6

RECIPES

Eating chicken breasts and broccoli every day is pretty healthy, but it gets boring pretty damn quick. Now remember, we're more concerned with fuel than flavor, but these recipes should help you out.

Besides having multiple things to choose from, you can also cook the same thing in different ways. Baked vs pan or boiled vs grilled.

We're going to kick this recipes list off with one of my all-time favorite go-to foods, tuna! I have been asked many times how I make it, so here it is. Aside from the mayonnaise, it's a pretty healthy meal/snack to have.

BENNE'S FAMOUS TUNA

INGREDIENTS:

- (4) 5oz cans of tuna
- (4) tbsp mayonnaise
- (1/2) cup dill relish
- (1/2) cup chopped white onion
- (4) chopped hard boiled eggs

PREPARATION:

- In a large mixing bowl or container, mix the onion and dill relish together
- Next, drain and rinse the 4 cans of tuna, then add them to the bowl
- Add the mayonnaise and mix until all the tuna is covered
- Let sit for about 5 mins, then add the chopped hard boiled eggs. Salt and pepper to taste

Can be eaten by itself, on crackers, on sandwiches, or any other way you can think of.

TURKEY PATTIES

INGREDIENTS:

- (1/2) lb 93% lean ground turkey
- (1/4) cup chopped onion
- (1) chopped garlic clove
- (1) tsp garlic salt
- (1) tsp Italian seasoning (basil, oregano, rosemary, thyme)

PREPARATION:

- In a large mixing bowl or container, mix all the ingredients
- Next, prepare a hot pan with a dash of olive oil
- Mold mixture into patty, thicker on the edges
- Cook both sides until dark and caramelized

Serve with a heaping portion of vegetables or black beans. Can also be served on a bed of brown rice.

PAN SEARED CHICKEN BREAST

INGREDIENTS:

- (1) large chicken breast
- (1/2) tbsp of butter or olive oil
- (1/2) tsp seasoning salt
- (1) tsp garlic powder
- (1) tsp onion powder

PREPARATION:

- Butterfly chicken breast
- Season both sides with mentions seasonings
- Add butter or olive oil into hot pan
- Sear both sides on med-high heat until caramelized
- Lower heat and cover until inside is cooked

Served with vegetables or with a side of brown rice. Also goes well when topped with sautéed onions or mushrooms.

SEARED SALMON

INGREDIENTS:

- (1) 6oz salmon fillet
- (1/2) lemon
- (1) tbsp olive oil
- (1/2) tsp lemon pepper

PREPARATION:

- Coat fillet with olive oil and evenly sprinkle lemon pepper on both sides
- Place into hot pan on medium heat for 3 mins, then turn and cook other side for 5 mins
- Remove fillet and plate. Squeeze lemon on the fillet

Serve with brown rice and light vegetables, such as squash or zucchini.

EASY GOURMET BREAKFAST

INGREDIENTS:

- (5) eggs
- (1/4) cup onion
- (1) chopped garlic clove
- (1) tsp pesto

PREPARATION:

- In a medium skillet, add onion and garlic into pan with a dash of olive oil. Cook for about 4 mins or until brown

- Add in pesto and mix with onion and garlic

- Pour in 5 scrambled eggs and cook until desired consistency

Serve with a slice of toast or a piece of fruit. You can also add chopped chicken or any other leftover protein you may have.

STIR FRY

INGREDIENTS:

- (1) cup chopped chicken or beef in 1 inch cubes

- (2) cups chopped broccoli

- (1/2) chopped carrots

- (1) tbsp olive oil

- (1/2) tsp garlic salt

- (1/2) tsp ginger powder

PREPARATION:

- In a hot pan, pour in olive oil and let sit until hot

- Stir in meat and seasoning. Cook for about 4 minutes, or until about halfway cooked

- Add in carrots and broccoli and cover. Lower heat to simmer and let sit until vegetables are tinder

Serve on plate and can add soy sauce if diet allows. Can also be served with brown rice.

BACHELOR BOWL

INGREDIENTS:

- (1/2) lb ground turkey (93%)
- (1) can black beans
- (1/4) cup chopped onions

PREPARATION:

- In a hot pan, put in turkey and onions
- Season as desired (ex: garlic, salt, pepper, oregano)
- Cook for about 10 minutes then drain meat
- Stir in drained can of black beans. Cover and sit for 5 minutes

Serve in a bowl. This is a quick an easy way to get a good meal packed with protein.

CHAPTER 7

FINAL THOUGHTS

This should be everything you need to get your plan started. Some people are a lot more strict with theirs and others not so much. It all depends on what your goal is. But whatever your goal is, suck it up, and demolish that shit.

Food and bodybuilding play a big part in getting a better, bigger, leaner body. The mind plays an even bigger role. Without having the mental focus and discipline, none of this matters. You need to look in the mirror and ask yourself if this is what you really want.

That mindset goes with anything in life. If you want it bad enough, then you will go out there and get it. It doesn't matter if you are just starting out or if you have been doing it for years, keep your eyes on the goal. You will have people along the way tell you that you can't or that you're wasting your time, don't listen. This isn't their goal and this isn't their dream.

If you happen to lose yourself along the way, pause, gather our thoughts and get back on the train. Ignore the nay-sayers because this is about you. Don't wait for a specific date or a certain time to start attacking your goal, start right now. Decide what you want, make a fucking plan, and work on that shit every single day.

If it doesn't challenge you, then it won't change you.